Book Of Treatment (Therapy) And Prevention (Prophylaxis) Of Anemia Made Very Simple For You

Olatundun Solomon

olatundunsolomon@gmail.com

Anemia is formed from the combination of two words, which are an and emia(an + emia) (an plus emia)(an +emia = anemia).

An is derived from Greek.

The meaning of an is lacking. The meaning of lacking is not having enough.

While emia is derived from Greek, which means blood condition.

Therefore, the meaning of anemia is blood condition whereby the blood is not enough.

Etiology Of Anemia

(Cause Of Anemia)

Etiology is from Greek word aitiologia meaning giving a reason for.

There are things that can make the blood condition in the body to not be enough.

Cause of anemia are:

1. Accident: Accident can cause trauma (injury). The injury can result to blood loss. The blood loss can make the level of blood to be low(anemia).

2. Decrease In Red Blood Cell Production.

When there is decrease in red blood cell production, it can result to anemia. Red blood cell is known as erythrocyte.

Erythrocyte is the combination of two words which are erythro and cyte(erythro+cyte).

The meaning of erythro is redness while cyte is cell. Therefore, erythrocyte is red blood cell. Erythrocyte (red blood cell) is produced from the bone marrow. The bone marrow is located inside the bone. But when there is cancer of the bone, it can cause the red blood cells to not be produced enough. This can cause anemia.

There can be decrease in red blood cell production when there is malnutrition(abnormal nutrition).

3. Iron deficiency:

Iron deficiency can also cause decrease in the production of red blood cells.

Iron is stored in the hemoglobin. It is needed for the production of hemoglobin. Hemoglobin is red pigment that carry oxygen in the blood to various tissues and organs of the body. It also carry carbondioxide from various tissues and organs out of the body.

Foods that contain iron that can be eaten are

Spinach,

Liver,

Shellfish,

Beef,

Turkey and

Legumes.

4. Vitamin B12 deficiency.

Vitamin B12 deficiency can also cause decrease in the blood that is in the body.

Foods that contain vitamin B12 are:

beef,

fish,

cheese.

milk and

eggs.

5. A diet that is frequently eaten that is low in folate, iron and vitamin B-12 can result to anemia.

Foods that contains folate (folic acid)(vitamin B9) are:

Dark green leafy vegetables such as broccoli, spinach, cucumber and lettuce.

Beans,

Liver,

Fresh fruits,

Whole grains and

Peanuts.

6. Thalassemia:

Thalassemia can also cause anemia. When thalassemia occur, there is faulty hemoglobin production. The name is coined from the Greek word thalassa this means sea. This is because thalassemia was first described in people that are living near the Mediterranean Sea.

The meaning of thalass is sea while emia refer to the blood condition.

Thalass + emia = Thalassemia.

7. Bone marrow tumor can also cause decrease blood production. This is because blood is produced from the bone marrow.

Hemogenesis is the combination of two words which are hemo and genesis(hemo+genesis=hemogenesis)

hemo refer to blood cells while genesis refer to formation. Therefore, hemogenesis is the formation of blood cells from the bone marrow.

When there is cancer of the bone, it can cause production of blood to be abnormal, this can cause the production of blood to be low which can result to anemia.

8. Malaria

Malaria can also make anemia to occur. This is because, malaria parasite (plasmodium) infect red blood cells (RBCs). The infected red blood cell lyses(break down).

The word lyses is from -lys- which means to break down.

The more red blood cell is infected and the more lyses (break down) occur, it will result to reduction of the blood level. This can result to anemia.

9. Hookworms (Necator americanus and Ancylostoma duodenale) stays in the small intestine of the body after infection. They attach to the villi of the small intestine and feed on blood. The loss of blood can result in anaemia.

Small Intestine villi:

Plural form is villi while singular form is villus, are small, finger-like projections that extend into the lumen(opening of the small intestine).

Hookworm infection is transmitted by walking barefoot on contaminated soil. The larvae penetrate the skin, and enter into the body. Hookworm (Ancylostoma duodenale) can be transmitted through the ingestion of larvae that is in contaminated food and water. It then attach to the villi of the small intestine and feed on blood. It is expected to drink clean water and eat well cooked food in order to prevent hookworm infection.

9. Whipworm:

Whipworm infection, also known as trichuriasis. The large intestine is infected by the parasite Trichuris trichiura. This parasite is known as whipworm because it looks like a whip. It feeds on blood. This can make the blood level to be low and result to anemia.

Whipworm can be transmitted into the body through bare foot from contaminated soil. And also by ingestion (swallow into the mouth) from water and food. It is expected to eat well cooked food and drink clean water to prevent it.

10. Ulcer:

When there is ulcer, ulcer simply means sore that feels like burning effect. This can occur in the stomach (gastric ulcer). Gastric refer to the stomach. Therefore, gastric ulcer is stomach ulcer. In stomach ulcer, there is sore on the lining of the stomach. This sore can cause blood loss and blood can be seen in the feces. This can result to low blood level (anemia).

Signs And Symptoms Of Anemia

Signs and symptoms of anemia are:

1. Pale Skin(Pallor).

Pale skin occur because of the reduction of red blood cells in the body. This is because hemoglobin (red pigment of the red blood cell) is decreased due to the red blood cells are reduced. The normal skin (cutis) becomes pale in appearance.

2. Jaundice.

Jaundice is a condition whereby the skin turn yellow in color. Occurring from excess of the pigment bilirubin produced by the liver in the body due to abnormal breakdown of red blood cells.

Hemolytic anemia(Hemo+lytic anemia) (Red Blood Cell+break down anemia) can cause it during malaria. During malaria, the malaria parasite (plasmodium) affect the red blood cell and break it down. The longer the parasite continue to stay in the blood, it will continue to infect more red blood cells and break them down. This is why the broken down red blood cells makes the bilirubin produced by the liver to be too much. Then it result to jaundice.

3. Excessive Thirst(Polydipsia): Polydipsia is formed from the combination of two words which are poly and dipsia (poly + dipsia). The meaning of poly is excessive while dipsia is thirst. Therefore, Polydipsia is excessive thirst.

There is increase in thirst. This is because there is reduction in the blood and it leads to low blood level(anemia). Because there is low blood level(anemia), this means there is low blood volume (hypovolemia)(hypo+vol+emia)(low+volume+blood condition)(low blood volume). When the blood volume is low it means that the fluid level of the body is low. This makes thirst to occur. This means dehydration has occurred. Dehydration (De + hydration)(removal + water) removal of water) due to removal of blood which become low(anemia).

4. Fatigue (Weakness).

Weakness occur because glucose (sugar) level of the blood is low (hypoglycemia)(hypo + glycemia)(low + blood sugar). It is the glucose in the blood that is used by the body as energy. The less the glucose (sugar) of the blood becomes, the more weak the body becomes because there is low level of energy.

5. Confusion:

It can cause confusion because the nutrients and glucose that nourishes the brain is low due to low level of blood (anemia).

Therapy Of Anemia (Treatment Of Anemia):

The treatment of anemia depends on the cause of anemia.

The drug(chemo-)(pharmaco-) that is used for the treatment of anemia is anti-anemic drug.

This is chemotherapy (pharmacotherapy). Chemotherapy is the combination of two words which are chemo and therapy (chemo + therapy)(drug + treatment). Therefore, chemotherapy of anemia is drug treatment of anemia.

Pharmacotherapy is the combination of two words, which are pharmaco and therapy. (pharmaco + therapy)(drug + treatment). Therefore, pharmacotherapy of anemia is drug treatment of anemia.

The drug treatment of anemia is anti-anemic drug.

Prophylaxis Of Anemia (Prevention Of Anemia):

Anemia can be prevented by eating foods such as:

Carbohydrates e.g wheat, yam, potatoes and brown rice.

Protein foods are beef, beans, chicken, turkey meat and goat meat.

Vitamins and minerals are in fruits and vegetables.

Oil can be found in peanuts, cashew nuts and also there are vegetable oils.

It is also expected to drink clean water.

Foods that contain iron that can be eaten are

Spinach,

Liver,

Shellfish,

Beef,

Turkey and

Legumes.

Foods that contains vitamin B12 are:

beef,

fish,

cheese.

milk and

eggs.

Foods that contain folate (folic acid)(vitamin B9) are:

Dark green leafy vegetables such as broccoli, spinach, cucumber and lettuce.

Beans,

Liver,

Fresh fruits,

Whole grains and

Peanuts.

Exercise is good for the body. It makes the bones to be strong and makes the body healthy.

When the bones are healthy and the body is healthy. Red Blood Cells (RBCs) can be produced from the bone marrow that can be enough for the body normal health. And thereby preventing anemia.